Sally Sharp
The Silent Authoress

By

Patty Polasky

Published by AuthorHouse 07/07/2022

ISBN: 978-0-7596-8591-8 (sc)
ISBN: 978-0-7596-8590-1 (e)

Print information available on the last page.

This book is printed on acid free paper.

Preface

Sally Sharp, The Silent Authoress
by Patty Polasky

This book is dedicated to all the women who have been physically, psychologically, and verbally abused by a spouse.

As one views the cultures of some Third World countries, one finds the women of some cultures have few rights. They may suffer beatings in public for even small infractions such as the exposure of part of their face for only a small moment. Frequently, women are denied the right to an education. There is only one reason a women in some Third World cultures is needed, and that is to procreate.

American women are not denied an education. However, sometimes within a marriage they may be denied further education as even in our society today the career of the husband (head of household) is stressed.

In the 21st century, this is a mistake because the husband and wife should share the advantages of extra schooling or career enrichment.

Countless divorced women have paid a huge price for educating a spouse. Frequently, a woman is left to endure the hardships and abuse because financially she cannot support her children with meager child support payments. So, year after year, she is forced to suffer physical, psychological, and verbal abuse. In addition, she frequently must hear how "worthless" she is as she is told this over and over by her spouse.

Deep within herself, she knows that once upon a time she won a college scholarship. She remembers always seeing her name listed on the Dean's Honor Roll List. She remembers all the offices she held in college, and she remembers even playing a movie star in the high school junior play!

Sally Sharp distinctly remembers that her father taught her to stand tall and use her brainpower to deal with life's challenges.

The message that Sally Sharp wishes to convey is "Get Out of the Abusive Situation." Find a way to leave. Have a rainy day fund for that purpose. Tell a family member or friend. Don't be afraid! Remember, you live in the United States of America. You are a person in your own right. Don't lose sight of all your accomplishments prior to being married. Have faith in your own ability to solve problems.

SYNOPSIS

SALLY SHARP by Patty Polasky

The story begins with a brief summary of Sally Sharp's life before she met Tom Sharp.

Sally works to help Tom through medical school and his Specialist Medical Degree (Radiologic Technology). While working Sally was leaving her young children to work to support the household. (This was frowned upon years ago, but Sally thought she was doing the right thing.)

With their children, Sally and Tom move to another city in order for Tom to set up his medical practice. Shortly after their arrival, Tom begins to co-author a book. He works earnestly for eighteen months on writing the material. Three weeks before the material is to be mailed to the publishing company, Tom tells Sally he needs X-rays, and she will have to be his guinea pig as he secures the necessary X-rays. It turns out to be 127 X-rays in a three week period.

The first night of taking the X-rays, Tom discovers Sally has a medical problem, but he doesn't tell her. Instead of telling her, he is sitting outside the doctor's office every time she goes to the doctor and anxiously awaits the news as to whether the doctor has discovered her problem. (The radiation swept her off her feet, as she was constantly going to doctors.)

Sally goes into detail on the traumatic experiences of being X-rayed over and over again. She describes the head and skull and facial bone positions and the hours spent on the X-ray table while her so-called loving husband stands behind a lead door!

After the taking of the X-rays, Tom starts to treat Sally very badly and later is out drinking every night, while Sally sits home with three children and a full-time job. In addition, she is very frightened by his presence. There is no crisis shelter for women.

At the time of the divorce, the judge hears the testimony of Sally's plight under an X-ray machine. Her case is heard by a three-man jury. (The judge, her attorney and Tom Sharp's attorney.) Her case is kept open because of the radiation she received.

Twenty months after her divorce, Sally discovers her medical problem as she suffers a fall at her home and has to be x-rayed at the hospital.

On the cover of the book to be published, Sally asks the question, "If the roles had been reversed, would the story have the same ending?'

Chapter I
Sally's Early Life Through College Senior

My name is Sally Sharp. I was the youngest child in a Catholic family.

We lived in a valley that was surrounded by some mountains in the state of Colorado.

My parents owned a large farm. We had horses, sheep, cows and chickens. The farmland produced various crops.

My memory of a very large garden is still etched in my mind. I remember in addition to potatoes, we planted green beans, peas, carrots, tomatoes, and other vegetables. In addition to our large vegetables garden, we also had another garden where watermelons and cantaloupe grew. We also had grapevines and plum trees.

My parents provided well for our family. It was always a delight to pass by the rows and rows of grapevines, especially when the grapes were ready to be picked. You guessed it! I tasted and ate some of them as I picked them from the vines!

As a child I vividly remember beef butchering day. My brothers and father conducted the ordeal. This was a mainstay of our food for the winter. In addition, we also would have preserved venison and pork.

Living on a farm in the summertime is a delightful experience. I distinctly remember playing school with all my dolls under the mulberry tree.

The mulberry tree was very large and provided much shade. I frequently ate mulberries from the big tree, even if they had not been washed. Sprays to get rid of insects could not be found on our farm, when I was a child.

I had pet hens that would sit on my lap. One really leery moment was when I realized my pet hen had laid an egg in my lap!

My brother, nearest to my age, was five years older than I. His name is Henry. Henry and I shared many wonderful experiences such as gathering the eggs, feeding the chickens, and putting out fresh water for them.

As Henry grew older, he helped with milking the cows. I never learned to milk cows. I always looked up to Henry and my oldest brother Clifford for their ability to do many different jobs.

My family planted a variety of crops. Harvest time was really a tense time as extra men would be hired to run the threshing machine to cut wheat.

My job included helping to prepare food for the hired men, my father, and two brothers (Henry and Clifford, who was 10 years older than I).

I vividly remember the large roasters and large kettles that we would use for cooking. This meant peeling many potatoes to provide mashed potatoes for the harvesters.

It was always necessary to provide lots of meat or poultry for the men as they would spend long, long hours in the field.

A man from the local creamery would pick up the cream twice a week. This meant that the milk would be put in a separator. I usually had to turn the handle of the separator as the milk was separated to produce cream.

As I grew older, I was taught the procedure for washing the separator. This was not one of my favorite jobs, because the parts of the separator were large and bulky.

Our family received a considerable amount of money from the cream we sold and at times large containers of milk would fill the creamery truck.

My family also received income from the crops we planted such as wheat and corn. The members of our family were always very industrious. They never hesitated to do menial jobs for other people in the community and usually were paid for their services.

Our family suffered greatly when my mother died from natural causes when I was nine years old.

As I was growing up, I learned to appreciate all the little things. I learned to value the importance of family. I also learned to appreciate the knowledge I was receiving through grade school. I learned to excel. I became very competitive and usually tried to make the highest grade in my class.

Singing in a trio was a highlight of my life, when I was an eighth grade student. I vividly remember singing solo parts as our trio performed during the Midnight Mass. Our church congregation sat silently as we bellowed out "Oh, Holy Night" and other Christmas hymns and carols.

I graduated from the eighth grade with honors.

I entered the public high school near the city where I had lived for years. I truly have always enjoyed being a student. However, I'm sure I had some anxious moments during those first weeks of being a high school student. I quickly realized I had to get my priorities straight and complete my work on time. I was thankful that I had been taught good work habits at my previous school.

I dearly loved my freshman year of high school. I even was runner-up for track queen. I played in the school band and sang in the chorus. Wearing a band uniform or special chorus outfit was always thrilling.

There were sad times during my freshman year of high school. My brother Clifford was drafted into the Army. This was during Word War II.

My father had waited a whole year and finally he received a letter from my brother. He was in a far-off land in the South Pacific.

During the war gasoline was rationed. I remember tires, sugar, and other items that were rationed.

My sister, Ada, had gone to work in an airplane factory.

At night my dad, brother Henry, and I would huddle around the radio and listen intently for the latest news regarding the war efforts.

My father encouraged me to get good grades and participate in extra-curricular activities. During my sophomore year of high school, I was runner-up for basketball queen. I also continued to play in the band and sing in the chorus.

A highlight of my sophomore year was getting a part in the junior three-act play.

As my sophomore year was ending, I had attracted the attention of one of the most popular guys in high school. He was a star football player. Sadly, his birthday was in late September, and he would be 18 years old.

Consequently, in late August he joined the U.S. Navy. Otherwise, he would have been drafted into the Army. His name was Kenny. He would have been a senior in high school. To this day I still have a spot in my heart for Kenny.

The vast majority of high school girls in my era did not engage in pre-marital sex. There were no birth control pills, and a terrible stigma was attached to having an illegitimate child.

I had a strong family foundation. We respected the rights of each other. All my Dad had to do was give me "That Look" by simply flashing his dark blue eyes to show his unhappiness. He never said a word, but I knew when he meant "No."

My junior year of high school was really an awakening. I was honored to be elected secretary of our Student Council and Editor-in-Chief of our high school newspaper.

I received numerous other honors. I continued to play in the school band and sang in the school chorus. A highlight of my junior year in high school was performing as a movie star in the school play. Our drama teacher even provided me with one of her elegant suits and high-heeled shoes to wear during the performance of our three-act play.

I had many friends as a high school student. I was always very competitive and took pride in being at the top of my class scholastically. My dad was very supportive.

My brother Clifford had come back from overseas because he had been injured in action. (He was injured while getting in a "fox hole".) Consequently, he was sent to San Francisco General Hospital for several months and then given a leave before receiving another assignment. Words cannot express the joy we shared when he came home.

One year and three months after our nation was attacked at Pearl Harbor by the Japanese, my brother Clifford was sent overseas. Later, he told us that there were 7,000 soldiers on the ship. His ship went through the Panama Canal and then traveled to islands in the South Pacific.

My brother Clifford will always be cherished. I know he went through "hell" during World War II.

In my senior year of high school I continued to excel in all my subjects. I was a twirler in our school band. I continued to work on the school newspaper. I had the part of a movie director in our senior play.

Upon graduation I was awarded an academic scholarship. My dad was very happy that I had received the scholarship and received the honor during graduation ceremonies. My classmates had voted me "Most Likely to Succeed."

College was a completely different experience. (I'm sure everyone who reads this story can identify with the overwhelming experience college presents.)

After a short adjustment period, I learned to budget my time and put my priorities in order. I continued to be listed on the Dean's Honor Roll and received several awards.

In my sophomore year I was voted Vice-President of the Student Council and Treasurer of the drama club. I also was listed on the Dean's Honor Roll.

My college honors continued through my junior year of college.

During the summer of my senior year, I took education classes and was given a provisional certificate. Our state had a severe shortage of teachers. Consequently, I signed a contract to begin teaching.

Why am I telling you (the reader) about my early life, home life, and education prior to meeting my future husband, Tom Sharp?

The answer is simple: I was reared in a loving family. We trusted our neighbors. We valued our clergymen, policemen, and educators. We felt complete safety within our homes and cities. We never locked our doors to our homes or cars. The Golden Rule was indeed, "Do unto others as you would want others to do unto you!"

Chapter II
Sally Sharp, The Silent Authoress
by Patty Polasky

My name is Sally Sharp. This is not my real name, but for various reasons, I will speak of myself as Sally Sharp and my former husband Tom Sharp.

Tom and I met and married while we were in college. Tom had one year of college and I had completed my third year. Tom had served in the U.S. Navy for two years prior to attending college. We both had set our goals of graduating and establishing a family and all the other traditional American family customs.

I began my teaching after completing my third year of college and Tom began teaching after one year. We were both elementary teachers, with provisional teaching certificates.

I met Tom within a week after I had returned a fraternity pin to a navy ensign because he was called from his reserve status to active service at that time. He, whom I'll call Hugh, was a wonderful person who completed four years of college and two years of medical school; but smart me—who could wait two or three years for a navy pilot to return home! I thought I needed a companion right then, so that's where Tom Sharp enters my life.

We were finally married after a lengthy courtship. The night before my wedding, I wanted to call it off. My sister was in town and tried desperately to reach me. She was older and more knowledgeable in the ways of the world and she was opposed to the wedding. (Just three months after Tom and I met, my father suffered a stroke. Two days after he suffered the stroke, he felt better and talked with me. The last thing he told me was, "Please do not marry Tom

Sharp. He will never be able to provide for you and you will have a difficult life.")

At the time I thought, "How can life be so difficult when there are only two of us?"

The wedding went on, and I can remember so vividly my sister crying at the reception. She could see things that I couldn't see.

I had always been an honor student and scholarship winner. In both high school and college I had received many honors from class officers, editor of school newspaper, movie star in school play, student council officer, basketball queen runner-up, track queen runner-up, and the girl voted most likely to succeed out of my high school graduating class.

After the honeymoon, I realized I had made a mistake. It was a secret that I kept buried in my heart, never to utter to a living soul. I had come from a religious family background and was taught that once one marries, it is for eternity. Also, I was taught that it is my responsibility to hold a marriage together. So after the honeymoon Tom decided to go to Radiologic Technology School. He was to receive $100 per month for two years. Somehow I struggled through this ordeal, living in a basement apartment that even had flood waters come in several times.

After two years of on-the-job training, he was to take his state registry examination, which he passed.

About the time he graduated from the school of Radiologic Technology, I discovered I was pregnant. We were still trying to buy furniture, a new car, and I was trying to go to school evenings and weekends. I had inherited a large sum of money, which was being used for the necessities and educational expenses.

I graduated four months before my daughter was born. Tom still only had one year of college, and now at last he had passed the Radiologic Examination and was a registered technician.

A year after our daughter was born, Tom decided to go back to college and enroll in the pre-med program. His GI Bill had run out, so now he decided to go to college. The incentive was the large sum of money from my estate that he wanted to receive indirectly by furthering his education.

Reluctantly, I left my nine month old daughter with a babysitter and went back to full-time teaching. I never will forget the things that were said, such as: "How can she leave her baby?" This was 1958, and women didn't leave their children when they were babies. I remember feeling so guilty each day that I was at school.

As a wife willing to promote her husband's interests, I left my nine-month old baby to go back to teaching in order for Tom to go back to college and receive his undergraduate degree, which he did.

There was always a constant struggle to pay tuition and college expenses and provide babysitting for our daughter while I taught school. I tried to be a good mother and a good teacher and nearly drove myself to destruction. There were art shows and special events and the principal knew I had artistic ability. Therefore, I would always be assigned to do the bulletin boards and other projects when special events happened.

In addition to helping support the family through teaching, I also helped my husband Tom by doing his research papers and book reports. I did three book reports in one week and he received an A on each report. (Little did I realize that I should be furthering my education and working on my master's degree that I started the summer before our daughter was born [6 graduate hours].)

By now our daughter is five years old, my husband Tom had graduated from undergraduate school that May and would begin medical school in September. Later that summer I discovered I was pregnant. I can truthfully say I wasn't all that excited at the prospect, because delivery of our daughter had been a traumatic event. I honestly felt as though I were dying. Little did anyone know the cause of my terrible delivery until events happened which I will tell you about later.

When our son arrived, we discovered that he had allergy problems and was extremely sensitive to foods. This was not known until countless trips were made to the hospital. Every time it was vomiting and diarrhea, and the same question was asked by the hospital staff, "Are you here again? Which room would you like to try?" After 48 hospital trips and three pediatricians, I finally consulted an allergist. If I ever felt I had "hell on earth" it was those dreadful days of either sitting for two hours in a doctor's office or walking the floor to get Don settled and asleep.

All this was done while I was still trying to teach. Many a night I would walk the floor all night long and stand on my feet and teach all day. Through this ordeal I was trying to help Tom through his medical school.

In January before Tom received his Medical Degree in Radiologic Technology, Jimmy was born. Jimmy too, suffered allergy problems, so there was the need for constant medical attention by the allergist. Now, there were two children with allergy problems, and the income wasn't that great. (Medicine and doctor bills are never free.)

In June, after Tom received his Medical Degree, it was decided that we should try to relocate to a drier climate because of our asthmatic children's health.

My two allergic sons continued to be sick all summer, and it was an immense, almost impossible ordeal to keep them out of the hospital. I spent two days a week at the doctor's office waiting for their shots and to be seen by the allergist. Then, night after night I was up all night long. I remember going all day and all night for six days straight, and the seventh day I hired a babysitter for several hours so I could go to sleep. I probably set a Guiness world record.

All summer, nearly everyday, and sometimes twice a day, it was necessary to get the house in order to show it off to someone who wanted to buy it. Then, there was the usual open house every Sunday. This was certainly a chore in view of the children always being sick.

There were countless other problems, such as knowing what to move and what to sell before the van came to move us.

Finally, the day came for us to move. We had made a trip in June to the city we chose. However, we did not have a place to move to directly, so we stored our furniture until we could rent a house.

Arriving in the new city with three children, a U-Haul and very little money, we rented a one-room motel with kitchen. We stayed in this motel for two weeks and finally were able to rent a house.

In spite of having a very small child, I applied for a teaching job and began my teaching career again. It seemed I only stopped long enough to have a baby and shortly thereafter I'd have to be back in the classroom, because we always needed the money.

After years of marriage, it was more than ever necessary that I return to teaching. I must admit that very, very often I felt guilty about being in the classroom, but somehow, to hold things together financially, it always was a must that I teach.

There was the need to get established in an office. There was equipment to purchase and office supplies, salaries, etc. There was always the need for bows and arrows, boats, lapidary equipment, rocks and gem stones and all the unessential things of life, when it came to the material things that made Tom happy on his time off.

I came from a family that had much pride and dignity, and no matter what the burdens were, I was taught to carry on and perform my duties as a wife and a mother with no complaints.

My own mother had died when I was nine years old. I had older brothers and sisters. However, I had learned at a very young age self-discipline. Along with self-discipline, I had a very competitive nature within me. (My honors continued through the years we were married and lived back in the east.)

Prior to moving to the desert and in spite of ill children, I was elected to serve on a college advisory Board of Regents. I had been past-president of my alumni association and had been active in my sorority.

To sum it up, when arriving in the desert city and faced with sick children part of the time (their health had shown drastic improvement living in the desert), and, of course, a small baby to care for in addition to my teaching job, it was impossible to be active in community affairs. Tom was always hollering about my new friends, but I felt overwhelmed with my role as wife, mother, teacher, homemaker and a million other things.

Shortly after our arrival, it was decided that Tom would author a book on Radiotechnology. For 18 months there was much attention devoted to writing the material that would become the manuscript. Some attention was given to securing x-rays to show how the human body actually looks, and the positions necessary to secure a particular kind of X-ray.

Having been taught to promote the interest of my husband, I became very excited about the fact that Tom was to author a book. "That was like getting your name on a marquee," I thought. Only, much to my surprise, one month before the book was to go to the publishing company, did I <u>find out</u> the role <u>I</u> was to play in the publishing of the Radiologic Technology book. I was told by Tom, my husband, that some X-rays using the X-ray machine and securing the real X-rays to be used in the book were to be taken of me. I was to be the victim receiving the radiation from these X-rays. (Back several years, while living in the other city, Tom became violently angry. From that night on I was extremely afraid of my husband.)

So, when the deal of being X-rayed came up, I was shocked and I <u>did</u> rebel, but then that terrible expression came over Tom's face like the night he became violently angry back in the east.

What a shock! Here I was to be someone's ever-loving wife, who had used a great percentage of my estate for his schooling, only to realize that I was being used such as you might use a mop to scrub a surface. I was no longer a wife. I was no longer a human being. I was only a guinea pig, because with only three weeks left to find the desired X-rays, there wasn't time to look through outdated films at the hospital. I was the chosen one to provide the real X-rays.

In the course of three weeks, 127 X-rays were taken at the local hospital and at his office. The X-rays were taken from 9:00 p.m. until 4:00a.m. at the hospital. At his office the X-rays were taken when the office was closed.

My husband, Tom Sharp, was the Radiologist taking the X-rays of his wife. He was the specialist. I was the guinea pig.

The first night 24 X-rays of the hip and pelvis were taken. I could have screamed when at 2:00 in the morning an accident victim came in and he had to stop X-raying me momentarily.

I put up a big fuss about being X-rayed and the radiation I was receiving. Tom thought he knew all the answers as he was a Radiologist. I was only a teacher that didn't know much about radiation. Repeatedly I was told there is no danger associated with taking X-rays. The old expression, "People have accidents every day and receive lots of X-rays." Little did I know that the first night I arrived at 9:00 p.m. and we were leaving at 4:00 a.m. with 24 X-rays of the pelvis and the hips. (These 24 X-rays the first night play a very important part in a later development in this story.)

I will always hate this part of my life. I felt I was absolutely stuck in a situation with a husband and a family. If I refused to be X-rayed, there would be drastic things taking place. If I consented against my will, I would suffer the consequences and be the silent authoress, with the children and no money and no place to go. There wasn't any choice!

As I laid on the X-ray table the first night the thought went through my mind, "I surely wish I could get up and call someone." I thought, "Tom is not playing fair. He's abusing my body for the sake of a book. Me! The mother of <u>his</u> children."

Tom Sharp had much difficulty getting the spinal positions as well as the sinuses, adnoids and facial bones. The X-rays had to be exactly correct. So many views were repeated. However, the material and X-rays for the book were finally assembled and airmailed to a publishing company.

Before the material even arrived at its destination, I was treated very badly. This continued and within one month after I had literally almost been swept off my feet by the radiation, I was told by Tom Sharp, my husband, "You aren't like other women, you can't go here and you can't do this—I'm going to bars, you've made me unhappy for years." Little did he know what radiation does to a person's body! I was completely and totally exhausted.

Within two days after the last X-rays of the facial bones were taken I vowed I would never again be subjected to this kind of abuse.

Before I got on the X-ray table prior to the first X-rays being taken, I said to my husband, "How can you do this to someone you love?" His answer, "I have no one else to X-ray!"

I must say after my role as silent authoress, I had much difficulty teaching. I was so extremely tired.

I had a wonderful babysitter. I told her all about the X-rays and she couldn't imagine someone using their wife for the sake of a book.

In the meantime, the months following the taking of the X-rays seemed to immediately change our lives. I never once mentioned the radiation I received to my husband Tom: but I found I was going to the eye specialist, internal medicine doctor, orthopedic doctor, and others. Nearly every trip I found my husband waiting in the office. Never once could I mention the radiation I received because that would trigger disaster. Teaching school, caring for a young child and two other children, plus being extremely tired was my thanks to the radiation I received. I didn't know until much later that people actually take off a year after chemotherapy treatments. In the two years that followed, I was treated very badly.

In September of the year that the book came off the press, Tom started drinking and staying out night after night. I his wife, was someone he literally hated. After nine months of night after night of sitting at home alone and waiting until he got home to lock the door (his arrival might be 1:00, 3:00 or 5:00 a.m.); and then I had to get up and go to my teaching job, while he came home drunk and was spending all the family money.

My sister died in the spring of the year that I filed for a divorce in June. When I went back to the east coast to my sister's funeral and realized that people went to bed at night, spouses were nice to each other, there wasn't any worry of money that I was experiencing, well I knew it was just a matter of a short time and I would file for divorce. At this time, none of my family knew about the X-rays and my part of being an authoress.

I tried to persuade Tom to go with me to a marriage counselor, but he told me, "You have the problems, I don't."

It had been a terrible struggle living through those last months from September through June. In analyzing my marital situation, I can only say I could count only five Medical Association dinners and one additional potluck dinner that I attended with my husband in the 9 month period. I felt that he knowingly took me to these functions where he wanted all his co-workers to know that he is that wonderful person they worked with every day. As for me, I felt like screaming out at those dinners that I, the wife of Tom Sharp, was married to the biggest damn heel there that night. My only bit of confidence building that I acquired at these functions were the comments made by some of the male co-workers (other doctors) at the dinners. Their comments personally were, "You really look nice tonight, Sally.", or "You are a very attractive person, Sally." Smiling, I would sip my drink and wonder, "Will I ever get out of this mess?"

Each day was an almost miracle day to survive. I never knew whether I'd have $5 to buy groceries for a week for five people or not.

I read all kinds of articles on alcoholism. I constantly was seeking advice or a clue as to how to handle the problem.

In May as I was going off to my teaching job, with my children going with me to their various schools or baby sitter and leaving by way of the front door, I passed our den each morning to find Tom stretched out with his clothes on and knocked out and snoring away! At this point I didn't care whether he lost his status as a Doctor of Medicine. He was nothing but a jellyfish to me!

For years I had struggled to see him through school and to always appease him by letting him get his way in whatever he wished to purchase or whatever he wished to do. It was constant sacrificing, and all my estate money had gone to his schooling. So when he was stretched out on the den divan and couldn't get up because he probably had only been to bed for three or four hours or less, well, I could care less. Through his drinking and wild spending, we were on the brink of losing everything we owned.

It's very difficult to realize that I had a college education myself and yet in order to preserve the family unity, I stayed and stayed in the marriage situation.

Something Dreadful happened the night before I filed for divorce that I was not permitted to say in court because the exact motive was not known for Tom's throwing boxes and papers in our garage. I'm not free to elaborate on this topic. All I can say is, that without hesitation, I filed for a divorce the next day.

The legal document was prepared. I was called to come sign it. I hesitated for only a second. Suddenly all the unhappiness of being afraid of the man I married flashed through my mind. I thought, "I'm attractive. Why should I sit waiting for him to come home at 3or 4 O'clock in the morning (every morning)? Am I to be a doormat to be walked on all my life? Is he to load me with radiation and then see if he can kill me through his wild behavior and complete lack of respect for his family and children?" I thought, "I'm a human being with dignity and self-esteem. No one will put me in a mental institution, ever!" So I signed the legal document. There was no choice.

The turmoil continued. For instance, Tom called my home at 2:30 p.m. on an extremely hot day to tell me that all the utilities were in his name and that they would be turned off at 5:00 p.m. So using the money received from a small insurance policy that came because I was the beneficiary listed on it from my deceased sister, I paid the utilities and deposits for my name to be listed on them. The deposits and utilities totaled $167 and the insurance money amounted to $500. Also, July 1st came and went, and, remember, I had filed for a divorce on June 20 (my husband had 20 days to respond). No child support was received on July 1st and for 10 days after. On July 10 my attorney received an answer to the legal document that Tom Sharp was served with on June 20. My attorney states, "Get some money to your wife and children before I'll talk with you." This made my husband angry. He brought $200 over and then acquires an attorney to defend him and to see that he will get his one-half interest!

On July 20 I appeared in court to establish child support payments. I was awarded $350 for three children. The division of property will be settled later.

My attorney advised me to get the exact amount of dollars and cents that we owe to various creditors, so I presented this to my attorney.

Several months passed before, I went over the divorce proceedings with my attorney. He explained about the financial statement, the assets, the debt, the amount needed for child support, and then he said, "We'll go over your case as the judge will present it in the courtroom." My lawyer said, "You will be sworn in and Tom Sharp will also be sworn to tell the truth." Then my lawyer friend followed: "State the reasons for this divorce." I answered, "Number one, the radiation I received from the X-rays my husband took so he could co-author a book on Radiologic Technology." My lawyer's comment, "Well Mrs. Sharp, you never said a thing about this before."

My lawyer wanted to know what book, how many X-rays, kinds of X-rays and everything associated with this.

I left the lawyer's office praying that night that there wouldn't be enough time on the judge's agenda the next day. Then I wouldn't have to go to court. Fortunately, there wasn't enough time because of too many criminal cases, so our divorce case was postponed.

On that eventful day, my lawyer called a blood specialist and sought other medical experts' advice. It was the common medical opinion that I should seek advice and be examined by a blood specialist. So an appointment was set up with that specialist. I never will forget the expression on the doctor's face (I'll call him Dr. Baker).

After telling the doctor that I was a human Guinea pig for my husband so he could co-author a book on Radiologic Technology, he said, "Who authorized the 127 X-rays?" I said, "My husband didn't get medical authorization from any doctor. He just took them. The first night he took 24 hip and pelvis X-rays from 9:00 p.m. to 4:00 a.m." But my husband is an X-ray technologist and Doctor of Radiology."

Blood samples were taken and sent to a special laboratory in another large city. Frantically, I waited for the report. A few days later I was called to come to the doctor's office for a report to be given by the doctor. I was told, "Sally, you have foreign cells in your blood." I cried and cried and only wished I had those trips to the hospital and doctor's office to live over again. I would not, under any circumstances be a guinea pig so my husband could have good X-rays while he stood behind a lead door making sure he received no radiation. This was my husband's thanks for all his education and training.

My father had taught me to stand tall and walk with dignity no matter what kind of problems I was to face. I walked out of that specialist's office realizing that I had been walked on by Tom Sharp, my former husband, but I was <u>not</u> <u>dead</u>! I vowed I would face reality. I would face future blood tests and pray with all my heart that I could live. I vowed I would rise above all my grief.

As if a Guardian Angel came down, suddenly I said to myself, "I will rise above my grief. I will go to court and I will tell my case to the judge exactly as it is."

Some months passed before our case came up in court again. Then, it was postponed again for various reasons. Almost thirteen months after I had filed for a divorce, our case finally came to court for final settlement. I had decided through the advice received from my lawyer that I would bring the charges of receiving the radiation of 127 X-rays in a three week period to the court room for the judge to hear. (Within two months prior to going to court, I had been called twice by my husband to "drop the stupid X-ray charges.") I couldn't stand to look at the book. However, I took it to court with copies of the royalties of Tom Sharp's part this edition. Part two involved the reading of a four page medical report by the judge and my description of the trips to the doctor's office, and the hospital for the 127 X-rays taken in a three week period. I described to the judge that we arrived at the hospital for the 127 X-rays at 9:00 p.m. (Twenty-four X-rays of the hip and pelvis were taken.) Two days later on Sunday morning we were at my husband's office taking X-rays and so forth. I stated in court to the judge, "Tom Sharp asked me to get on the table under the X-ray machine, and I said to him, "Tom Sharp, how can you X-ray me and give me this radiation if you love me?" His answer was, "but I have no one else to X-ray!" I continued telling the judge, "The last night was absolutely terrible. I had my facial bones, sinuses and adnoids X-rayed over and over again. I felt my head would actually break. I vowed I would never permit myself to be X-rayed one more trip not one more X-ray. I could not look at one more sandbag."

Tom Sharp first had said he only took a few X-rays. In court he said he took 35 X-rays, but he didn't know how many more because he didn't keep track!

In view of the fact that there was no medical reason for me to have these X-rays, and, undoubtedly, there was more than a few, the judge ruled our divorce case be kept open. The judge granted the paying of $1.00 a year alimony.

Prior to the judge's awarding of the alimony, Tom Sharp's attorney questioned me as to why I permitted the X-rays to be taken. I said, "Because Tom Sharp was violently angry back in April 1968, and I've been extremely afraid of him ever since." Tom Sharp's attorney stated, "No more questions asked." The judge said, "Divorce granted."

Having been taught divorces are experiences only to people who can't work out their differences, I realized I had an impossible partner. My divorce was a struggle for survival. Someone had to take command of the ship. There were two minor children at home to love and cherish.

Following my divorce I went back to school and received my Master's Degree in Public School Administration. Also, I took a modeling course which helped to reestablish my self-confidence.

Twenty months after the divorce was granted, I fell at my home one evening. I was in absolute, excrutiating pain; but not having the $42 cash for an ambulance call, I struggled to my bed and had a terrible agonizing night.

The next morning my good friend, a lady I taught with, took me to the local hospital emergency room. My son had had a foot injury the year before, so we had crutches at home, and I used those to get myself to the emergency room.

At the emergency room I was X-rayed and absolutely screamed and screamed with pain. There I was told that I injured old injuries and would be on crutches for a while. I was also advised to go to an orthopedic doctor the next week.

My visit with the orthopedic doctor was really a jolt. I was told I reinjured old injuries that I received in a car accident. I discovered that I had a fractured hip, a dislodged hip, a pelvis broken in two places and crushed in another. Then the doctor said, "You have had absolute miracle babies. How did you ever live through the birth of three children?"

I cried when told of my injuries and the need for hip surgery eventually. But the doctor said, "You are very fortunate, Sally. Four-and-one-half years ago nothing could be done for your hip problem. Now there is surgery to correct it."

I went home from the doctor's office feeling very sad and blue. Suddenly, I realized why my ex-husband was always sitting outside the doctor's offices when I visited them during those last three years of marriage before I filed for divorce.

I couldn't imagine Tom Sharp treating me so badly, then worrying whether there was anything wrong with me! I thought perhaps he thought I'd say something to the doctors about the radiation I received from the X-rays. My report from the orthopedic doctor gave me the exact reason I was treated so badly by Tom Sharp.

The first night of taking the X-rays he told me he had trouble getting a good left hip X-ray. He had discovered that I had a hip problem, and who wants a wife with a problem like that? How could someone go through medical school and not know where the hip socket is located? I had told my friend numerous times that there was something mysterious surrounding those X-rays.

Yes, there was something mysterious. That mystery was solved when I was told of my old injuries by the orthopedic doctor. My ever-loving ex-husband could not only load my with radiation, he could tell me to go to hell because I had a problem that he cause when he hit a truck in May 1955. (At the time, X-rays were taken, but I was told by the clinic I visited that I had no broken bones. I went back to teaching one week later with a purple leg!)

Yes, this is what one human being can do to another. To the person, the nearest and dearest to you, you can use, abuse and then start behaving badly by being critical and drinking and being out all hours of the night. After several years, a divorce situation had been created.

For me, the person that was used as guinea pig under an X-ray machine, criticized and belittled constantly, then told, "There's the front door. Go out whenever you wish, with whomever you choose." That was the response I got when I asked Tom, "Why don't we go out together tonight?"

One thing that my experience has taught me is that silence is not blessed when you are abused. I, the silent authoress, am no longer silent, because I am an authoress in my own right. I needed no one to assist me with this story.

In closing I will say to everyone, "Be strong, think positive thoughts, and remember you, too, can stand alone." To Tom Sharp I will say, "I hope and pray that I'm wise enough to choose a MAN the second time around, not a weak man that runs when a problem occurs."

There's an old adage, "Once burned, twice wise." If in the person, Tom Sharp, there was love (in our marriage) it certainly went out the window the night the hip and pelvis X-rays were taken for the book. But love is truly a mystery as I stand alone today. My many years of seeing him through all his advanced education and a zero balance from my inheritance, have indeed prompted much soul searching.

However, my regular trips to the blood specialist and my constant body check for radiation burns remind me of one thing. Never will I be abused by any man, nor will I ever be a silent authoress again, even if it is for the sake of a spouse getting his name on the cover of a book.

My two goals in life are to rear my two minor children and to write another book. So until then, goodbye, and God bless you.

Chapter III
Life After My Divorce

No one, absolutely no one, can tell a person what a tremendously challenging responsibility rearing two sons alone is without a family support system. My family lived over a thousand miles away.

The first year was traumatic in that money was so very difficult to manage, when support was so small and my job was not a high-paying job.

Many and many a night I felt so angry with myself in that I had trusted my children's father to provide for us, and I could quit working. Just as my father told me on his deathbed, "Don't marry Tom Sharp because he will never be able to provide for you." My father was very wise. Years later I wondered if what my father really meant was, "If Tom is successful in a career—down the road, he'll leave you and your kids. Consequently, he'll never provide for you."

At the time of my divorce, degrees secured by the father during the marriage were the father's possession and no financial compensation was given to the mother even though without her efforts financially, there would have been no degree or degrees.

It was not until 1981 that Sullivan versus Sullivan, a Supreme Court case, established the right of a spouse to demand and receive compensation for educating a spouse. The Women's Movement was ill-advised and left many women in distress. In many cases, the thought of being able to keep 100% of your earnings less meager child support actually created the possibility of divorce in some men's minds, as greed overcame compassion. A divorce can easily be created if a financial problem arises and it's easier to divorce than to deal with the financial problem with the marriage.

The security of a career is a godsend when one is divorced. I tried to be the very best teacher I could be and I tried to be a good mother. Many times that meant not getting much sleep because of my sons' asthma and allergy problems.

A divorce is a traumatic experience after a long marriage.

This chapter is being written 25 years after being granted a divorce. As I analyze my circumstances at the time of the divorce and the fact of seeking a divorce, I had no choice at the time. I asked my children's father twice to go for counseling, but his reply both times was, "I don't need counseling. You are the one who needs counseling." I kept my appointments with the counselor in spite of my children's father not being in attendance.

I was granted full custody of two minor children. I must admit there were times when I wasn't sure whether I could carry out my duties.

Three years after my divorce was granted, I was rear-ended in a car accident in which I suffered a brain concussion. This was a very difficult time, because I suffered severe headaches and was seen by a neurologist for one whole year on a bi-monthly appointment, with EGG performed at least once a month.

Six months after the accident, I was hospitalized for four days where I had the EGG wires attached to my head. As I remember, the neurologist felt this to be extremely necessary. To add to my problem, I knew immediately after the accident that I could not tell my principal that I was going for EGG tests or even give him any ideas that I couldn't perform my duties as a teacher.

Fourteen months after the accident, my doctor assured me that my brain had returned to normal.

I felt extremely lucky to be able to teach through the ordeal and still care for my sons.

My luck was short-lived as I was injured by a child with a disability, who had much difficulty walking.

I received a displaced vertebra injury. It took two years before I could sleep at night as previously. I would be awakened every time I turned my body in bed while sleeping.

I sought help from an acupuncturist as a last resort. The neurologist had told me there was no surgery to correct my problem. I was using crutches to walk and feeling extreme pain from the spinal injury.

It had really been an ordeal to teach school, care for my children, and try to keep my priorities focused.

There's an old adage, "God never gives you more that you can handle." That adage frequently crossed my mind. I prayed and prayed that I would recover from the spinal injury. My sons were very helpful, but trying to manage financially was the greatest worry.

One day, while recuperating after the spinal injury, I received a phone call from the secretary. She informed me that "today was my last sick day, and if I didn't appear for work tomorrow, I would be placed on medical leave with no salary."

There was no question. I must go back to teaching in the morning. I told the secretary I would be back the next day.

I was injured the week before Christmas vacation. I tried to come back for a day, but I had to go home. Consequently, I was out of school Christmas vacation and three weeks after Christmas vacation, but the spinal injury also caused severe injuries to my abdomen. My abdomen and related organs hurt so very badly. In fact, I thought I was going to die three different times following this injury.

Arriving home from teaching school all day, I would take a brief rest. The truth is, how could I rest, when I had two hungry boys that were starved. Therefore, the key was planning our meals. Never once did my sons complain about our meals.

I knew I had to protect their health. Therefore, I tried to provide wholesome meals. We seldom had TV dinners. We occasionally had fast food, but fast food is expensive so this rarely happened.

My sons grew up knowing what it was like to conserve food and money. I tried to provide the things they really felt were necessary. I remember purchasing a record player with stereo sound system for my elder son at Christmas. He had taken an interest in music and was playing an instrument in his middle school band.

My elder son was a Boy Scout. I felt I could not deny him the opportunity to participate in scout activities. It was a wonderful experience for him. He went on many scout trips and learned real-life experiences through his scout training. In addition, he received many badges and lacked only one badge from being an Eagle Scout.

I could write a book on working with your children to ensure their success. I always checked my younger son's homework. Many a night that meant reviewing his spelling word lists in preparation for a study. I distinctly remember helping him learn the multiplication tables, just as many parents help their children.

It is extremely important for parents to attend their children's conferences and know exactly what's happening in the classroom. It gives comfort to your child to know that you care. I was that kind of parent.

I tried to have my sons participate when invited to a classmate's birthday party, whether it was a private home or public restaurant. My sons also invited guests to our hme, or sometimes a party was arranged at a pizza or McDonald's restaurant. It is very important that our children have some fun time.

Rearing children as a single parent is extremely difficult. If a mother is taking nighttime college classes, the early morning hours provide a good time for studying for a test or completing term papers.

There were semesters when I was taking two 3-hour college credit classes, and one summer I spent the entire summer vacation attending college in order to complete my Master's Degree. Thank God for my elder son who cared for my younger son while I was attending college.

I began my Master's Degree 22 years earlier, receiving six graduate credits, and now I'm a single mother with two children to support! Also, I must acknowledge my deceased sister's (Meg's) foresight as she named me as a beneficiary on her insurance policy. In addition, I also received inheritance monies from my deceased sister Meg.

I was so short of money when I finished my Master's Degree, I passed up the opportunity to accept my degree in person because I did not have the money for a cap and gown—$28.00. I cried and cried, but I never told my sons the reason I wasn't attending my own graduation ceremony. I learned a bitter lesson by sacrificing so very much to put my children's father through years and years of school. I denied myself further education at the time.

No one, absolutely no one, gives credit to an ex-spouse for financially seeing them through until they reach their terminal degree. They have the education and "to Hell" with the Golden Rule—"Do unto others as you wish others to do unto you."

A single, formerly married mother's life changes so drastically once she is divorced.

The entire rearing of the children to a great extent is given to the person having primary custody. This necessitates much planning, particularly for food and clothing. I tried to shop at the supermarket once a week. I would spend every Sunday afternoon cooking. I would cook roasts, chicken, meatloaf, and other recipes. and usually double the recipe. My sons loved roasts with potatoes and carrots. I tried to vary the chicken recipes. We also had Hamburger and Tuna Helper later in the week. I prepared big bowls of vegetables and relishes.

The sacrifices that a former spouse has to make after a divorce from a person with a terminal degree are endless.

The "Macho commanding" position displayed by my children's father is forever etched in my mind.

Not being compensated for spending years of my life and much sacrificing to see a spouse through until he reached his terminal degree was extremely traumatic for me.

As I write this many years later, I truly believe in many cases the only love that existed in my marriage ended when handed the diploma at the commencement giving the spouse the terminal degree he wanted.

Everything in our marriage was according to my former spouse's demands. Many years there was not a penny for a vacation, even though I taught and everyone else was taking trips!

Women need to think in terms of making a legal contract if they are educating a spouse. I would suggest a formal binding legal contract drawn up by an attorney indicating compensation expected.

Even with Sullivan versus Sullivan court case 1981, women are still being excluded, if there is any possible way around it. In essence, a true partnership would mean that when one spouse gets a year of college, then the other spouse must get a year of college! But this seldom happens. Usually there are children and the expenses are too high.

Another way to look at leaving a spouse at the graduation ceremony is called being deceitful. <u>Very, very deceitful</u>. I firmly believe this happens in about 80% of cases where women educate a spouse.

As I look back on my life since I was abused under an X-ray machine, I would never permit a spouse to abuse me again.

Why did I permit this abuse to take place? The answer is simple: that I was frightened. I feared for my life. If one has never lived through this extreme fear, one will never know such a traumatic experience.

Firstly, I feared for my life and lived in fear two and a half years prior to the x-rays being taken.

An event happened that forever changed my life. That event was the night my children's father came home from an evening (10:00 p.m.) college class and was violently angry. Immediately he went to his closet to get the box that contained the razor-sharp arrows and also got his bow from the closet. Then he went to the phone book and looked up the instructor's name and address, wrote it down, and left. slamming the back door.

I was absolutely horrified. Then my children's father, Tom Sharp, began practicing his archery by shooting the arrows against our garage door.

Zing-Zing they went.

My neighbor called and asked what was going on at our house. I replied, "Tom is upset!"

As I was talking to my neighbor on the phone, Tom Sharp drove his car out of the driveway.

I will never forget that moment. I literally thought our name, his name, would be in dark headlines on the front page the next morning.

I called my friend and told her what was happening. Her husband got up, dressed, and went to find my children's father.

I had given my friend the instructor's name and address as Tom Sharp was hollering out the address as he was writing the name and address down. He was violently angry.

The night I had to experience the x-raying over and over again of my facial bones, I wanted to scream, "You bastard, why are you doing this to me, while you stand behind a lead door??"

I knew that fateful night, that I had to get out of the marriage. I had three children—and older child in high school and two younger children.

If I had to relive this ordeal again, I would flee after the first night of x-rays.

I would have called my sister Meg to send money. Then, during the day, I would have picked up the children at school after I had the car packed to leave. I would have taken some of the children's clothes and toys, as well as my personal belongings and clothes.

Silence is not blessed when one is abused.

Years later I can vividly remember those dreadful weeks following my abuse under an x-ray machine. I had absolutely no energy, yet I was a full-time teacher with thirty students to teach. I was the housekeeper, laundry lady, ironing lady, caretaker of young children, cook, and so called wife.

Never did I receive a "thank you" for receiving the radiation from the x-rays. Never was there a mention of the x-rays, but as previously stated, my former husband was outside the doctor's office every time I had a medical appointment.

My children never knew about the radiation I received until years later.

My daughter graduated from college after being married and having a baby. She graduated with honors.

As I look back years later, I remember the expectations my former spouse had. He told me, "We are going to the hospital, because I need to x-ray you for the book." I yelled, "But I'm not a guinea pig."

Instantly a terrible expression came over his face. I identified it to be the same fierce look he gave me the night he was going after his college professor with a bow and arrow!

I remember vividly his response to my unwillingness to be a guinea pig. His reply was "I have no one else to X-ray!"

I've tried not to dwell on this through the years, because mentally it could strip a person of their innermost strength. It could crush a person's ability to survive. In fact, experiencing this trauma at the hands of my spouse and then being verbally abused over and over again through the next three years caused great stress and grief. Yet I had the children to care for, which was overwhelming at times.

As I look back on these terrible years of my life, I can honestly say that I made the biggest mistake of my life when I didn't file for a divorce the day after he was searching for his college professor with a bow and arrow. This was several years prior to my being his guinea pig!

In my generation, women were taught to support their men. They were told to take a back seat to his demands. With due respect, many men of my generation showed kindness and love to their spouses. In many cases, they have remained married through the years.

My biggest regret in later years was not pursuing my terminal degree. I could easily have had a doctoral degree or law degree, as I was accepted at several universities for a Ph.D. program and I also was accepted as a law student at a prominent law school.

As a single divorced custodial mother, I tried to make certain that my sons graduated from college.

As I end this book, there's an old adage, "All good things come to those who wait."

Through the years, I received many honors and awards. However, some of my greatest achievements have come during the last five years.

I retired from teaching a year ago. I've been recognized for my intelligence and have met and communicated with some of the greatest minds on earth. In the end, I've used my skills to accomplish numerous goals.

To any woman who is in an abusive situation, I say, "Get out! if you don't leave, life will only get worse. Remember: You are a human being and you deserve to be treated fairly."

In closing, I could have married twice since my divorce. However, the bitter memories I have of being abused under an x-ray machine, warrant my choice to remain single.

Had crisis shelters been in existence at the time of my abuse, I'm, sure I would have chosen to leave the marriage much sooner.

Chapter IV
Trauma of Being Used Under an X-ray Machine

Moving to a new city was a devastating experience for me. Never once did I foresee being used under and x-ray machine as being part of Tom Sharp's plan to publish a book!

Tom felt as though he was on "Cloud Nine" after learning he was authoring a book.

Sometimes I would be at the grocery store at 10:00 at night or scrubbing the kitchen at midnight. There was always a mountain of work to do.

Tom continued to spend all of his free time on the manuscript and rarely helped at home.

I was also excited about the book. I remember asking Tom, "Could I do something to help you?" His reply was, "No, you wouldn't understand it."

The second summer after completing one year of private practice, Tom began to spend more time on the book.

Tom told me, "We have to have the material to the publishing company by the end of September."

I frequently felt I needed to be taking classes toward my master's degree. However, Tom would always come up with some reason for me to not get involved with classes, especially while he was co-authoring a medical book.

The weekend before my school teaching assignment began was always a hectic one. Friday evening of that weekend, shortly after finishing our evening meal, Tom informed me that I would be going with him.

Tom said, "You are going to the hospital with me tonight." Then he continued, "I need some x-rays for the book."

I vividly remember responding by saying, "I'm no guinea pig."

Then this violent facial expression appeared and he said, "Get ready!"

I wanted to cry and cry. I felt as though I was an animal being loaded in a truck to take somewhere.

I was very frightened, but the thoughts of the bow and razor-sharp arrows flashed through my mind.

I knew I had no choice not to submit to even one x-ray.

Why did I submit to the x-rays? I reasoned that Tom would probably kill me if I didn't submit to the taking of the x-rays.

Then, my thoughts flashed to the children. I would never want them to not have a mother; they were so young.

The trauma I experienced the first night of being x-rayed is forever etched in my mind.

Over and over my hips and pelvis were x-rayed (24 x-rays).

Traveling home, I could hardly stand to look at my husband. He had not given me one minute prior notice until he said, "We are going to the hospital. I need x-rays."

Tom's behavior was so strange on the way home and after arriving home, that I was afraid to go to sleep!

Tom was always cold-hearted. Never once did he tell me to go to bed and get some extra rest.

I was a very healthy person, and there was no medical reason to take x-rays. However, within two days after the x-rays were airmailed to the publishing company, Tom began to act as though he was unhappy. Often he wouldn't speak unless asked a question that he could give a yes or no answer.

I vividly remember the day after the last x-rays were taken. I was driving the car down a busy street and suddenly I felt electricity passing through my body from the top of my head to my feet. I thought I was dying.

Startled and shocked, I pulled to the side of the road. After the initial shock, I thought, "I must go to the police." But then Tom would lose his job, and what would happen to the children?

As I drove to my job, I thought, "Is this a warning from God?"

When I arrived at school there was no one to tell what had just happened to me. Also, what would my friends (coworkers) think of my stupidity in permitting the x-rays to be taken? My answer to the last question as, "They are not in my shoes. They are not living with a violent man, who has little regard for human life."

It was on that day as I was driving home that I vowed I would not be a guinea pig again.

Never once did Tom Sharp say, "I'll only need one more x-ray."

I was saved by a deadline he had to meet to get the material to the publishing company. (He had already gotten a one-week extension on the contract, and they told him they would not give him another extension.) Tom mailed the manuscript to the publishing company.

Sadly, I found out later that all of the x-rays could have been obtained form the outdated files at three local hospitals.

There were no women's crisis shelters at the time of my abuse. I had no relatives in the city where I lived. It is devastating to know that I was trapped by my own spouse.

Physically, the x-rays had made me very, very tired. I came home and absolutely couldn't get out of the rocking chair. Yet, my spouse would scream at me or shout at me that I wasn't like other women!

I remember thinking, "You may have a lot of knowledge about medicine, but you have no knowledge of what radiation does to the human body."

I wrote a letter to my sister, but I just put Dear ____. In essence, the letter said I was giving up my most previous possession, my health.

This was among the most traumatic times of my life. I was completely exhausted as I made appointments with various doctors. Never could I utter a word about being abused under an x-ray machine.

The radiation had depleted my energy, and the verbal abuse continued day after day. It's very difficult to be the ever-loving wife under these conditions.

As the next year passed, we attended five social functions. I was slim and tried even harder to be beautiful when I attended these formal social functions. Secretly, as I sipped my drink sitting by Tom Sharp, I thought, "I'm married to the biggest damn heel here tonight."

The two things that kept me going were my looks and brainpower. I knew I didn't have to be walked on because I was still very good looking and smart. I refused to think about the radiation I received. Had I dwelt on the fact of being x-rayed over and over again, I'm sure I would have ended up in a mental institution.

Many times I was in the classroom without any sleep. The trauma of not knowing what would happen from one day to the next was terrible. I knew I had been abused and often entertained the idea of a scheme to leave and flee with the children.

The death of my sister, Meg, was devastating. I regret that I never told Meg about the x-rays, but Meg knew how I was being treated. In fact, she was preparing a rental property she owned as a place for the children and me after I divorced Tom Sharp.

I spent a week back home and realized that spouses were kind to each other and people actually slept at night!

My Catholic religion had taught me to respect my husband and do everything in my power to keep our marriage intact. My children's father joined the Catholic Church only to marry me. He was not reared a Catholic.

Religion plays a big part in dealing with a spouse. I think young girls need to be taught that there are times when it is impossible to hold a marriage together.

I think young girls need to be taught that spousal abuse, whether physical, verbal, or mental, should not be tolerated.

How many Home Economics or Family Unity classes ever present steps to be taken if one is found in an abusive situation?

My ex-husband called several times before we went to divorce court and yelled at me to "drop those stupid x-ray charges!"

Had I not (at last) been firm in my conviction that I must proceed with the x-ray charges, I might have said, "I'll drop the charges."

The reality is that I would have permitted my former spouse (Tom Sharp) to abuse my body for the sake of a book.

Believe me, I had some frustrating times. One night I got so emotional I threw Tom's good red woolen sports jacket in the rosebushes at 1:00 am.

I was so upset that I cried and cried.

Then I remembered what Meg, my sister, said to me one time on the phone. "Do not throw Tom's clothes out on the street. The court will side with him and say you put him on the street."

Quickly, I retrieved the red woolen jacket and other articles of clothing I had thrown into the bushes.

Shame plays a big part when one is contemplating a divorce. I as the first and last family member to seek and be granted a divorce. This was the last thing I wanted for my children. I knew the trauma they would face for many years to come. In fact, our divorce was a scar, one that they would live with for the rest of their lives.

Educating a spouse and neglecting one's own advanced education is a very big mistake. I paid dearly financially for the rest of my life.

Even today women are still educating a spouse and if a divorce occurs, they will not have the financial means to support their children and themselves.

It's a very big mistake to continue with a marriage when the spouse doesn't want to go to counseling. I made the mistake of trying to "hold on" to the unrealistic concept of thinking that I could change my spouse's personality.

The longer one stays in a marriage after everything seems to be "falling apart" only makes for more grief. In my own case, I should have left the marriage after the zinging of razor-sharp arrows on our garage door back in the previous city. I had been extremely frightened, and this should have been a warning sign of things to come.

Immediately, I should have confided in my sister, Meg. She was 15 years older than I. If I had dealt with that event by facing the violent anger of my spouse with help from relatives or professional medical people, I might have avoided the potential problem of being x-rayed over and over for a book.

My advice to anyone reading this book is the following:

1. Try never to show verbal, physical, or mental abuse toward your spouse. IF you are

completely frustrated, leave the scene, even to step outside your home or dwelling.

2. Attend marital retreats or conferences.

3. If your spouse turns up with a health problem, research the problem and seek from medical professionals, not divorce attorneys.

4. Put a percentage of each check in a fund for a weekend or week's vacation without the children.

5. Cherish your mate. Keep your romance alive.

6. Be kind to each other. Remember, your spouse is "on loan" from God.

7. Lastly, never hurt your spouse by physical, mental, or verbal abuse.

Every day I live with the potential of a severe health problem. I've suffered by being told "you have leukemia, and we'll start treatment in one month." (Fortunately, God had another plan for me.) Later, a biopsy showed I had precancerous cells that necessitated immediate surgery.

In closing, to Tom Sharp, I would like to ask, "If the roles had been reversed, how would you feel, if you had been abused under an x-ray machine by your spouse?"

"How would you feel if you had educated your spouse and then received *zero financial compensation* for your efforts?"

"How would you feel if you had to spend the rest of your life worrying and coping with the effects of unnecessary radiation?"

These are questions that only Tom Sharp can answer.

As you read my story, remember that there were no women's crisis shelters in the city where we lived at the time I was abused under an x-ray machine.

In closing, I could have married twice since my divorce. However, the bitter memories I have being abused under an x-ray machine, warrant my choice to remain single.

Had crisis shelters been in existence at the time of my abuse, I'm sure I would have chosen to leave the marriage much sooner.

As I end this story, I would like to salute the men who remain loyal to their wives and who have no intentions of abusing them. God Bless All of You!

Also I end this story, I am grateful for having been awarded an academic college scholarship.

A year after my divorce, I enrolled in modeling school. I enjoyed modeling at fashion shows. I was even asked by the owner of the modeling agency to travel to New York City for a show seven years after first entering modeling school. I declined as I had a minor child at home.

During my years as a single divorced mother, I've had two other part-time jobs. Earning extra money was a necessity.

My master's degree was in public school administration, but that would mean many hours at school and working 11 months a year. Besides, the field had few women administrators at the time I would have been seeking a position.

As I look back on my life, being abused under an x-ray machine has been the most traumatic event of my life. To realize that I was trapped in a marriage with a spouse who didn't give a damn how much radiation I received, is still very difficult to comprehend.

Silence is not blessed when one is abused. I am no longer a <u>silent authoress.</u>

Patty Polasky grew up in the Midwest. She lived in a small town where her great grandparents and grandparents had settled in the 1850s. They came from Europe.

She vividly remembers her early childhood as being filled with many happy memories. Patty has said, "Growing up in a small town gives one a sense of security. The reality is that even our neighbors were considered part of the family!"

Patty went on to college where she majored in communications and education. She later obtained a Master's Degree in journalism.

She taught school for fifteen years, then decided to become a freelance writer. She has received numerous honors for her literary efforts in recent years.

Patty would like the readers of the book *Sally Sharp, The Silent Authoress* to know that some women experienced great hardships, especially during the early years of the women's movement.